My Mediterranean Salad

*50 Delicious Salad Recipes for Your Healthy &
Light Mediterranean Meals*

Jenna Violet

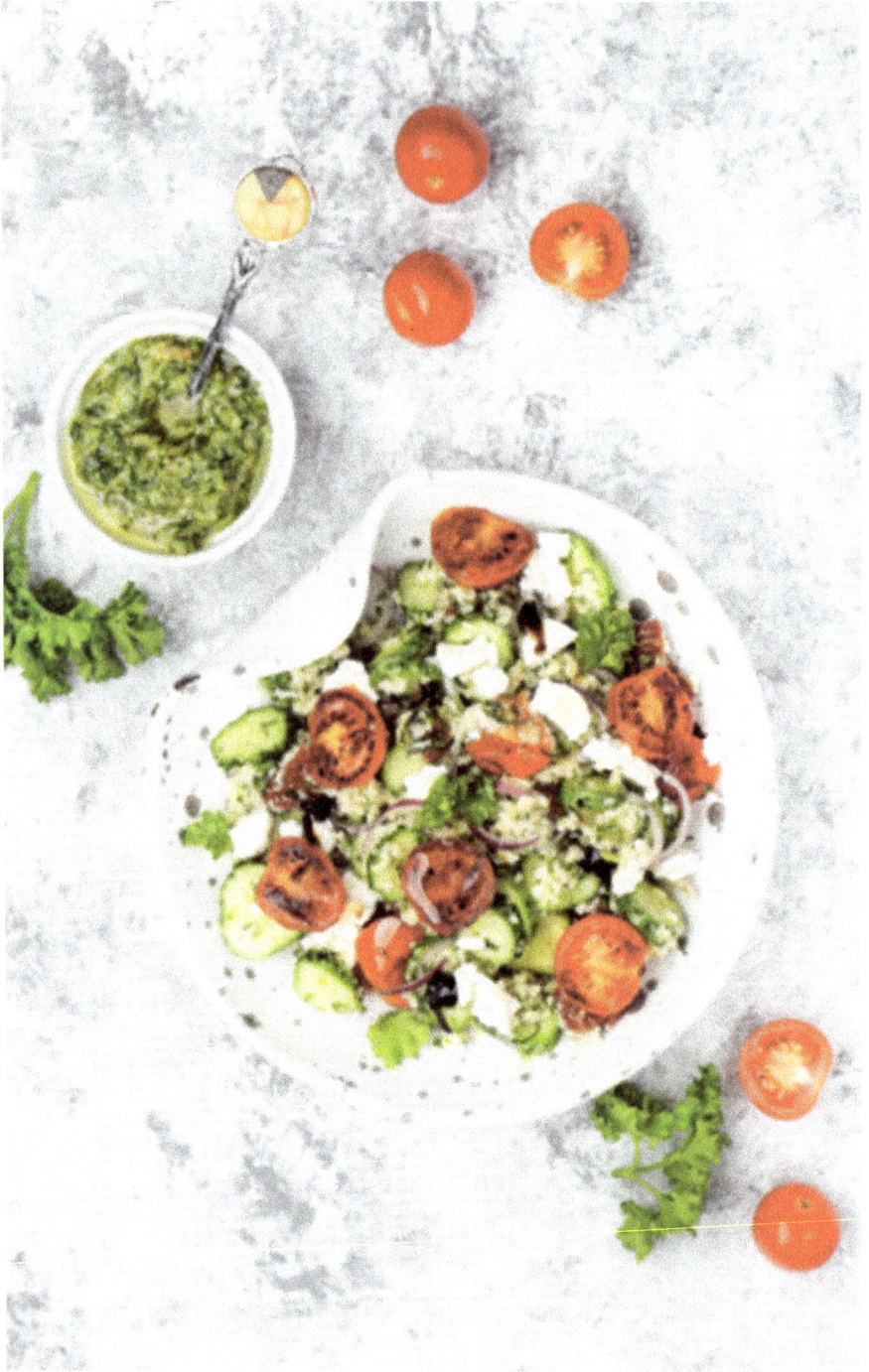

By reading this document, the reader agrees that under no circumstances is the author responsible for any losses, direct or indirect, which are incurred as a result of the use of information contained within this document, including, but not limited to, — errors, omissions, or inaccuracies.

Table of Contents

CHICK SALAD WITH LIMA BEANS, BEETS AND SPINACH 7

CREAMY POTATO AND HAM SALAD 9

CHICKEN AND CUCUMBER SALAD WITH PARSLEY 12

SHRIMP, ARUGULA, WHITE BEANS, CHERRY TOMATO SALAD 14

VEGAN CHOPPED CHICKPEA GREEK SALAD 17

MEDITERRANEAN PASTA SALAD 19

HORIATIKI SALATA 21

CHICKPEA AND SPINACH SALAD WITH AVOCADO 22

SPINACH, CHICKEN AND FETA SALAD 24

MEDITERRANEAN CHICKEN SALAD PITAS 27

HALIBUT WITH LEMON FENNEL SALAD 29

PITA SALAD WITH CUCUMBER, FENNEL, AND CHICKEN 31

ORZO VEGETABLE SALAD 33

BALSAMIC CUCUMBER SALAD 36

GREEK COUSCOUS SALAD 37

MEDITERRANEAN SHRIMP ORZO SALAD 39

ARUGULA AND WILD RICE SALAD 41

MASALA LENTIL SALAD WITH CUMIN ROASTED CARROTS 43

ROASTED AND RAW CARROT SALAD WITH AVOCADO 46

ORANGE ORZO SALAD WITH ALMOND, OLIVES, AND FETA 49

CRUNCHY THAI PEANUT QUINOA SALAD 52

COLORFUL VEGGIE LETTUCE WRAPS 54

CHICKEN BACON SALAD WITH HONEY MUSTARD DRESSING 57

DAD'S GREEK SALAD 59

TZATZIKI POTATO SALAD 61

MEDITERRANEAN COBB SALAD 63

NECTARINE AND BEET SALAD 65

BALSAMIC CUCUMBER SALAD 67

TZATZIKI SHRIMP CUCUMBER ROUNDS 68

TOMATO FETA SALAD 70

CHERRY TOMATO SALAD 72

GREEK SALAD DRESSING 74

GARDEN TOMATO SALAD 76

WHITE BEAN SALAD 78

3-INGREDIENT MEDITERRANEAN SALAD 80

TRADITIONAL GREEK SALAD 81

MEDITERRANEAN WATERMELON SALAD 83

MEDITERRANEAN CHICKPEA SALAD 85

CHICKEN SHARWARMA SALAD BOWLS 88

MEDITERRANEAN COUSCOUS SALAD 91

MEDITERRANEAN CAULIFLOWER SALAD 94

WATERMELON CUPS 97

SIMPLE GREEN JUICE 99

MIXED BEERY SMOOTHIE 100

APPLE PEAR GINGER SMOOTHIE 101

DETOX GREEN JUICE 102

MATCHA ICED TEA 104

MEDITERRANEAN GREEN SALAD 106

STRAWBERRY SALAD WITH POPPY SEEDS DRESSING 108

Chick salad with lima beans, beets and spinach

This recipe is crunchy, sweet with a vibrant color packed with fiber, mineral, and vitamins. It also serves as a great appetizer for a dull meal.

Ingredients

- 2 tablespoons of unsalted butter
- 5 radishes
- 2 chicken breasts
- 2 beets
- Salt and pepper
- 1 cup of fresh lima beans
- 1 can of sweetcorn
- 4 cups of fresh spinach

Directions

- Place in a large pot and fill with water.
- Bring to the boil.
- Lower the heat after 40 minutes of boiling and let simmer for another 10 minutes.
- Drain any excess water and allow it to cool.
- Shell the pods.

- Slice the radishes, put in a bowl together with spinach.
- Next, slice your chicken breast into thin strips.
- Season with salt.
- Melt butter in a frying pan.
- Place the chicken strips in the pan, let fry until golden brown.
- Add the lima beans together with the sweetcorn.
- Sauté for 3 minutes.
- Season with black pepper.
- Serve and enjoy.

Creamy potato and ham salad

Ingredients

- 1 lb. potatoes
- Black pepper
- 2 carrots, medium
- 5 ounces of dill pickles
- 4 medium eggs
- 2 teaspoons of salt
- ½ cup of mayonnaise
- 1 onion, medium
- 5 ounces of canned peas
- ¼ cup of sour cream
- 5 ounces of ham

Directions

- Clean and peel the potatoes and carrots.
- Place them in a pot.
- Add the eggs and pour in water.
- Add 2 teaspoons of salt, cover.
- Let the water boil. Lower the heat to let simmer for 10 minutes.

- Transfer the eggs into a bowl. Let cool in cold water.
- Let the potatoes and carrots continue to cook until done.
- Drain out any excess water, then chop the vegetables.
- Chop the onion, drain the peas.
- Drain and slice the dill pickles into small pieces and dice the ham.
- Peel the eggs, cut into small pieces.
- Move every content to a large dish. Mix properly.
- Add the potatoes with bit of salt and black pepper.
- Combine the mayonnaise with sour cream.
- Stir into the salad until well combined.
- Taste and adjust accordingly.
- Refrigerate for many hours preferably overnight.
- Serve and enjoy.

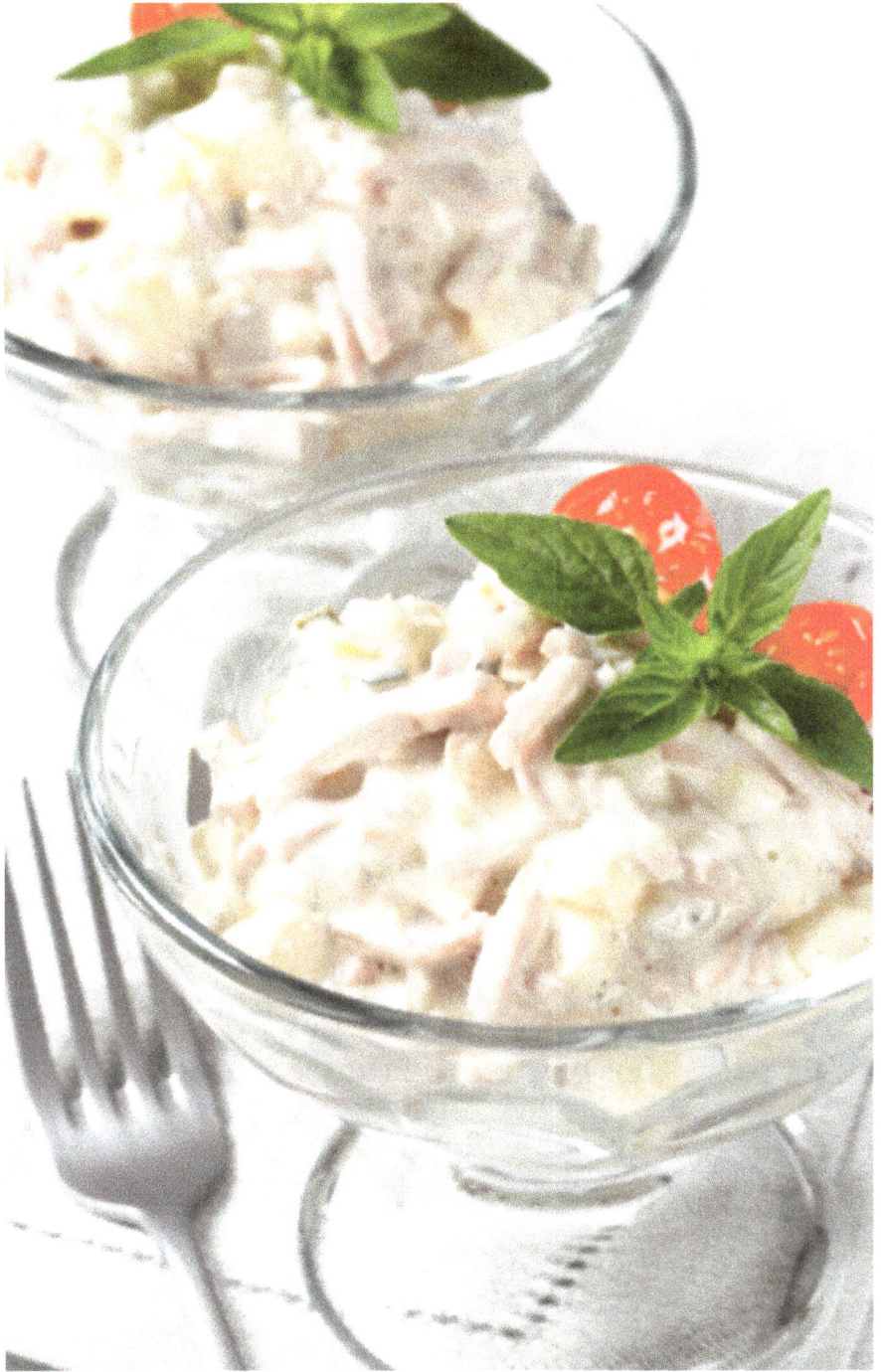

Chicken and cucumber salad with parsley

This recipe is like a powerhouse of protein mainly the chicken and chickpeas along with edamame. It gets ready only in 15 minutes making 6 servings

Ingredients

- 4 cups of loosely packed arugula
- 1 teaspoon of kosher salt
- 1 cup of fresh baby spinach
- 2 tablespoons of fresh lemon juice
- 1 tablespoon of grated Parmesan cheese
- 1 cup of chopped cucumber
- ¼ teaspoon of black pepper
- ½ cup of extra virgin olive oil
- 1 medium garlic clove, smashed
- 2 cups of packed fresh flat-leaf parsley leaves
- 4 cups of shredded rotisserie chicken
- 1 tablespoon of toasted pine nuts
- 2 cups of cooked shelled edamame
- 1 can of unsalted chickpeas, drained and rinsed

Directions

- Combine together parsley with spinach, cheese, pine nuts, garlic, lemon juice, salt, and pepper in the dish of a food processor.
- Blend or process until very smooth in 1 – 2 minutes.
- As the processor is still operating, add oil blend for 1 more minute.
- Stir chicken together with the chickpeas, edamame, and cucumber in a bowl or dish.
- Add pesto, toss.
- Put arugula in every bowl topping with the mixture of chicken.
- Serve and enjoy immediately.

Shrimp, arugula, white beans, cherry tomato salad

This recipe is made up of a massive combination of healthy and tasty vegetables making it a perfect tasty Mediterranean Sea recipe for a vegan.

Ingredients

- ¼ teaspoon of black pepper
- 1 cup of cherry tomatoes, halved or quartered
- ½ cup of finely diced red onion
- ¾ teaspoon of grated lemon zest
- 3 handfuls of baby arugula leaves
- 3 tablespoons of red wine vinegar
- 2 15-ounce cans of cannellini white beans, rinsed and drained
- 1 pound of 16-20 count shelled and deveined shrimp
- 2 cloves of minced garlic
- ½ teaspoon of salt
- 3 tablespoons of extra virgin olive oil

Directions

- Heat a large skillet over high heat.

- Add 2 teaspoons of olive oil to coat pan.
- In batches, add the shrimp, sauté for 1 minute on every side to sear when the oil is hot enough.
- Remove from pan when almost ready, keep to cool.
- Place drained beans, lemon zest, diced onion, cherry tomatoes, and arugula leaves into a large bowl.
- Fold in the shrimp.
- In another separate small bowl, whisk red wine vinegar together with the olive oil, garlic, salt, and pepper.
- Make a fold of the dressing into the salad.
- Serve and enjoy.

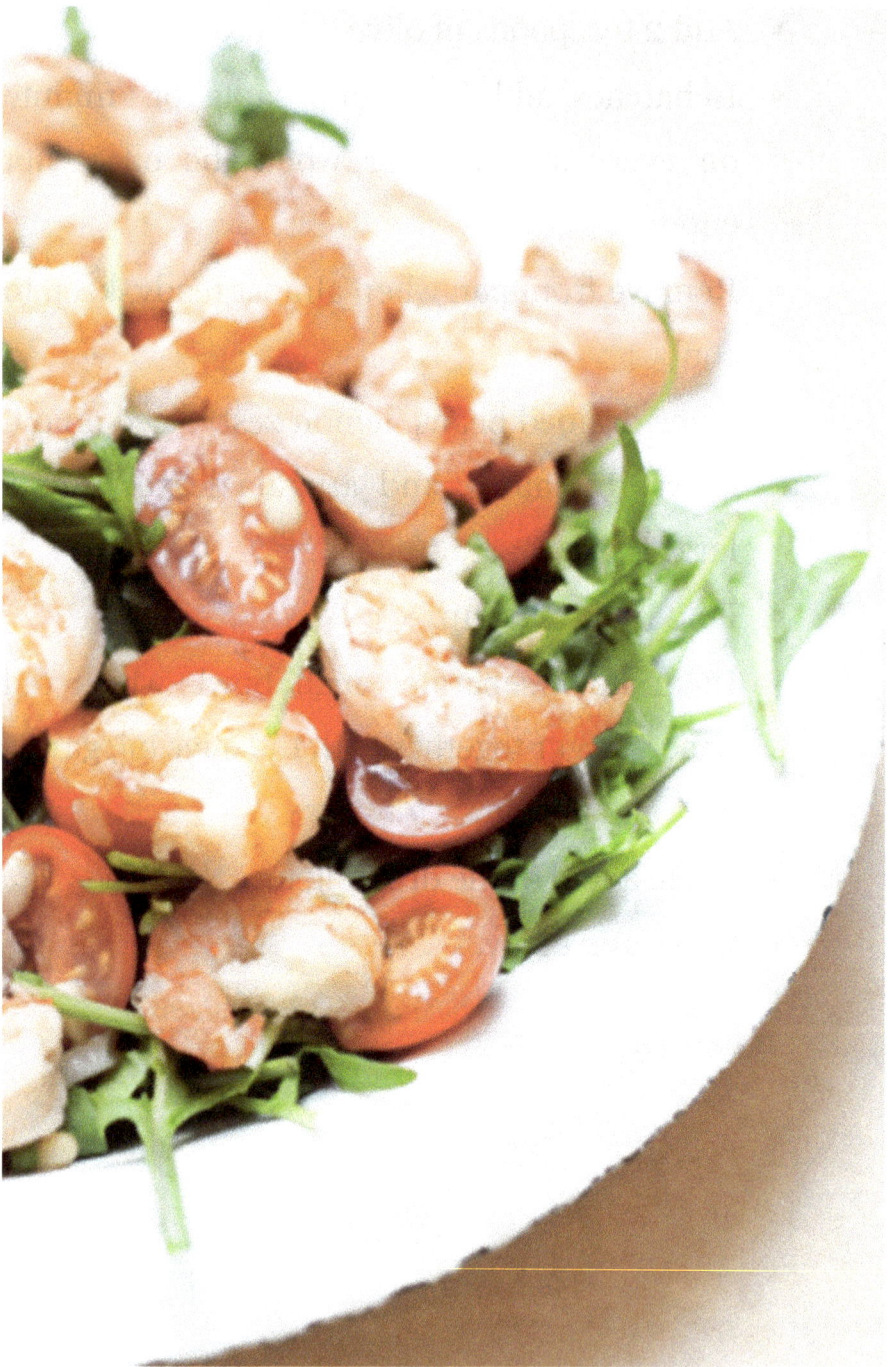

Vegan chopped chickpea Greek salad

Unlike other recipes, this vegan chopped chickpea Greek salad and other veggie salads does not need cooking at all. As a result, everything is prepared and consumed raw for a typical Mediterranean Sea vegan diet.

Ingredients

- 1 medium bell pepper thinly sliced
- 1 medium red onion thinly sliced
- 2 cups of cherry tomatoes halved
- 1 cup of black olives sliced
- 1 large avocado
- ¼ teaspoon of salt
- ¼ cup of olive oil
- ½ teaspoon of Italian seasoning
- 8 cups of baby spinach
- 3 teaspoon of balsamic vinegar
- 1 teaspoon of lemon juice
- 1 can of chickpeas drained and rinsed
- 1 teaspoon of honey or date syrup
- 1 large cucumber sliced
- 1 teaspoon of Dijon mustard

Directions

- First, add olive oil, vinegar, lemon juice, honey, Dijon mustard, and salt in a jar.
- Shake well to combine.
- Arrange all veggies and chickpeas on beds of spinach.
- Add avocado and dressing right.
- Serve and enjoy.

Mediterranean pasta salad

This pasta salad is a perfect meal for light lunch or dinner although it takes up to 4 hours to get ready. In a nutshell, patience is highly recommended.

Ingredients

- 1 teaspoon of kosher salt
- 1 ½ cup of crumbled feta cheese
- 1 pint of grape tomatoes, sliced in half
- ½ teaspoon of ground black pepper
- 1 cup of Kalamata olives, pitted, coarsely chopped
- 1 cup of green olives, pitted, coarsely chopped
- ½ red onion, diced
- 1 large cucumber, diced
- 5 ounces of hard salami, sliced
- 1 pound of dried fusilli
- 1/3 cup of olive oil
- 1/8 cup of balsamic vinegar
- 1 tablespoon of granulated sugar
- 2 cloves of garlic, finely minced

Directions

- Start by cooking pasta as directed on the package.
- Drain excess water and put in a large bowl.
- Add tomatoes, cucumber, olives, feta, red onion, and top with salami.
- In another separate small bowl, whisk olive oil with garlic, sugar, balsamic vinegar, salt, and pepper.
- Pour over pasta mixture, toss to coat.
- Refrigerate for 4 hours or more.
- Serve and enjoy when the time is up.

Horiatiki salata

Ingredients

- 1 large cucumber, peeled and sliced
- ½ teaspoon of oregano
- Splash of red wine vinegar
- ¼ red onion, cut into thin strips
- Salt and pepper
- 10 Kalamata olives
- 3 medium tomatoes, quartered
- 6 ounces of feta cheese
- ¼ cup of extra virgin olive oil
- ¼ red bell pepper, cut into thin strips

Directions

- Add all veggies together with the olives to a bowl.
- Top with olive oil, feta cheese, vinegar, and oregano.
- Add salt and pepper
- Serve and enjoy.

Chickpea and spinach salad with avocado

This meal makes a staple diet in the Mediterranean countries with variety of vegetables and herbs to give it a maximum flavor for lunch and dinner.

Ingredients

- 1 avocado, sliced
- 1 pound of fresh spinach
- 1 red pepper, chopped
- 3 tomatoes, chopped
- 1 bunch of fresh cilantro, chopped
- Salt and pepper
- ½ cup of extra virgin olive oil
- 1 onion, sliced
- 1 pound of boiled or canned chickpeas
- Balsamic vinegar
- 1 cup of mushrooms, sliced

Directions

- Together, put chickpeas with tomatoes, mushrooms, avocado, onion, red pepper, spinach, and cilantro in a mixing bowl.
- Add salt and pepper to your liking.

- Add olive oil together with the balsamic vinegar to taste.
- Mix and serve.
- Enjoy.

Spinach, chicken and feta salad

Ingredients

- 1 teaspoon of sugar
- 1 package of prewashed baby spinach
- 1 teaspoon of bottled minced garlic
- ½ teaspoon of salt
- 1 tablespoon of fresh lemon juice
- 1 teaspoon of Dijon mustard
- 1 teaspoon of olive oil
- ¼ cup of fat-free, chicken broth
- 1 can chickpeas drained
- 1 pound of skinless, boneless chicken breast
- ½ teaspoon of grated lemon rind
- ¼ teaspoon of black pepper
- Cooking spray
- 1 ½ cups of chopped red onion
- 1 tablespoon of balsamic vinegar
- 1 ¼ cups of pieces of yellow bell pepper
- ½ cup of crumbled feta cheese

Directions

- Combine chicken broth, lemon rind, lemon juice, vinegar, sugar, garlic, dijon mustard, olive oil, and salt in a bowl and whisk.
- Heat a large skillet coated after coating with cooking spray over medium-high heat.
- Sprinkle chicken with black pepper.
- Add chicken to pan let cook for 4 minutes, flip over.
- Add onions and cook for 4 more minutes. Make sure to stir frequently.
- Cut chicken into thick slices.
- Combine chicken together with the onion, cheese, bell pepper, chickpeas, and spinach in a large bowl.
- Drizzle with vinaigrette over salad and toss well.
- Serve and enjoy.

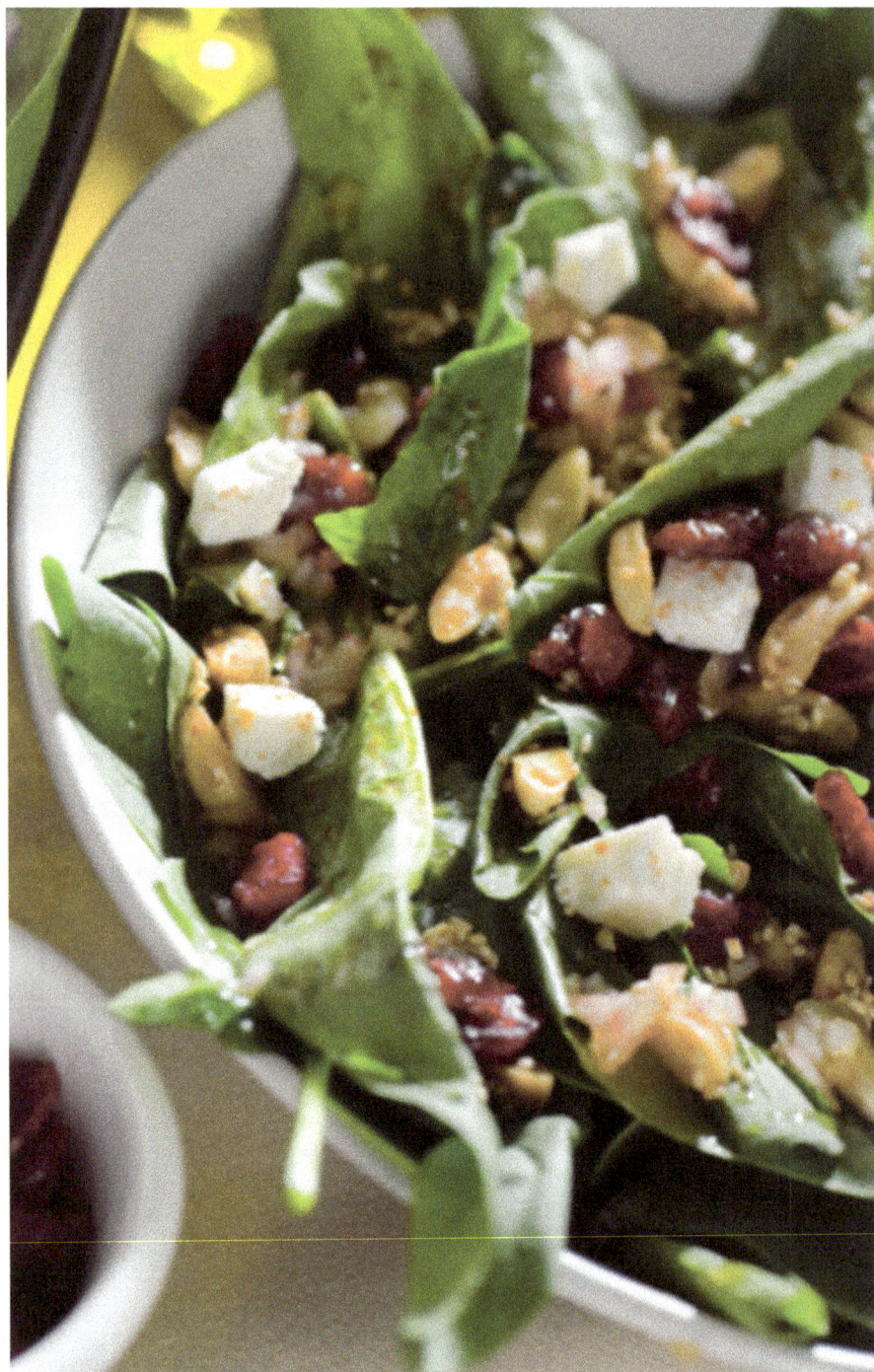

Mediterranean chicken salad pitas

No doubt everyone loves eating chicken; as such, this Mediterranean chicken salad pita comes in a new twist with greed thick yogurt. It also has a rich flavor consistence.

Ingredients

- ½ Teaspoon of ground cumin
- 6 slices of tomato, cut in half
- 3 cups of chopped cooked chicken
- ½ cup of chopped pitted green olives
- Cup of plain whole-milk Greek yogurt
- ½ cup of diced red onion
- ¼ cup of chopped fresh cilantro
- 1 can of chickpeas, rinsed and drained
- 2 tablespoons of lemon juice
- 6 whole wheat pitas, cut in half
- Cup of chopped red bell pepper
- 12 bib lettuce leaves
- ¼ teaspoon of crushed red pepper

Directions

- Combine the yogurt, lemon juice, cumin, and red pepper in a small mixing dish.
- Combine chicken together with bell pepper, green olives, red onion, cilantro, and chickpeas in another separate small mixing dish.
- Mix the two mixtures above and toss to coat.
- Line each pita half with 1 lettuce leaf and 1 tomato piece.
- Then, at least add ½ cup of chicken mixture to each pita half.
- Serve and enjoy.

Halibut with lemon fennel salad

Ingredients

- 1 teaspoon of fresh thyme leaves
- 1 tablespoon of chopped flat-leaf parsley
- ½ teaspoon of salt
- 5 teaspoons of extra-virgin olive oil, divided
- 4 halibut fillets
- 2 garlic cloves, minced
- 2 cups of thinly sliced fennel bulb.
- ¼ cup of thinly vertically sliced red onion
- ¼ teaspoon of freshly ground black pepper
- 1 teaspoon of ground coriander
- ½ teaspoon of ground cumin
- 2 tablespoons of fresh lemon juice

Directions

- In a small mixing bowl, combine coriander with salt, cumin, and black pepper.
- Then, combine the spice mixture with oil and garlic in a small bowl.
- Rub the garlic mixture evenly over fish.

- Next, heat a large skillet over medium-high heat with oil to coat.
- Add fish let cook for 5 minutes on every side.
- Combine the balance of the spice mixture with oil balance and fennel bulb., and all ingredients in a medium bowl and toss.
- Serve and enjoy salad with fish.

Pita salad with cucumber, fennel, and chicken

Ingredients

- 3 tablespoons of extra-virgin olive oil
- 2 cups of thinly sliced fennel bulb.
- ½ cucumber, halved lengthwise, sliced
- ½ cup of chopped fresh flat-leaf parsley
- 1 cup of shredded skinless, boneless rotisserie chicken breast
- ¼ teaspoon of black pepper, divided
- 2 pitas
- ¼ cup of fresh lemon juice
- 1 tablespoon of white wine vinegar
- ¼ cup of vertically sliced red onion
- ½ teaspoon of salt, divided
- ½ teaspoon of chopped fresh oregano

Directions

- Firstly, preheat your oven to 350°F.
- Organize your pitas on the baking sheet.
- Bake for 12 minutes and toast well.
- Let cool for 1 minute.

- Then, break them into bite-sized pieces.
- Combine pita pieces, fennel, together with chicken, parsley leaf, red onion, and cucumber in a dish.
- Sprinkle with salt and pepper to season to taste.
- Combine juice, oregano, vinegar, salt, and pepper in a bowl.
- Whisk with oil.
- Drizzle dressing over pita mixture and toss well.
- Serve immediately and enjoy.

Orzo vegetable salad

Orzo vegetable salad's taste and delicacy is elevated with the tangy lemon dressing over chilled orzo and whole vegetables. This vegetable recipe is a true Mediterranean Sea diet healthy for anyone and served along with any meal.

Ingredients

- ¼ teaspoon of pepper
- 3 plum of tomatoes, chopped
- 2 green onions, chopped
- 4 teaspoons of lemon juice
- 1 tablespoon minced fresh tarragon
- 2 teaspoons of grated lemon zest
- 1/3 cup of olive oil
- 1 cup of marinated artichoke hearts, chopped
- 1 cup of coarsely chopped fresh spinach
- ½ cup of crumbled feta cheese
- 2 teaspoons of rice vinegar
- 1 tablespoon of capers, drained
- ½ cup of uncooked orzo pasta
- ½ teaspoon of salt

Directions

- Begin by cooking the orzo as per package Directions.
- In a large bowl, combine artichokes, tomatoes, onions, spinach, cheese and capers.
- In another small bowl, whisk all dressing ingredients.
- Drain orzo and rinse.
- Then add to vegetable mixture.
- Pour dressing over salad, toss well.
- Allow it to chill.
- Serve and enjoy.

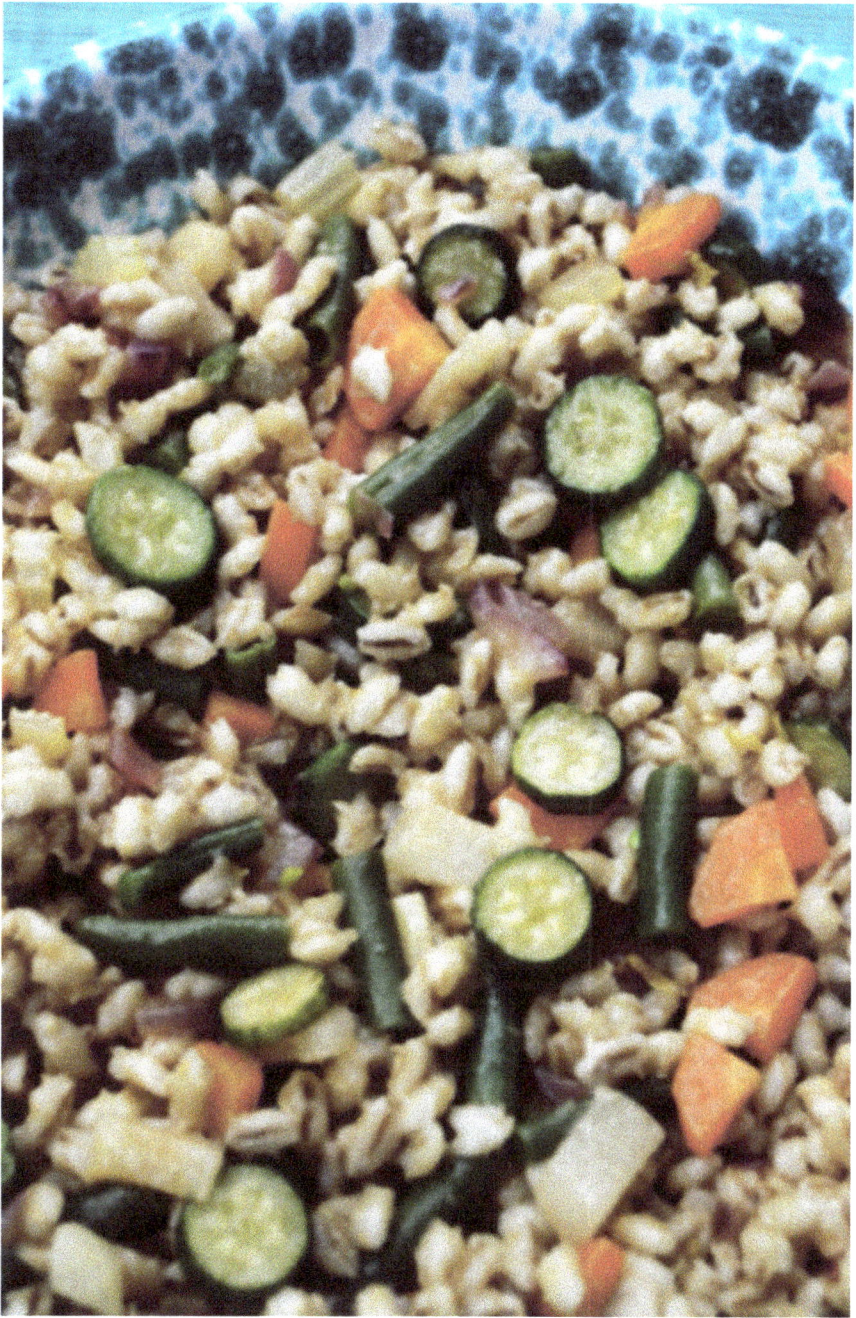

Balsamic cucumber salad

Ingredients

- ¾ cup crumbled reduced-fat feta cheese
- ½ cup balsamic vinaigrette
- 2 cups grape tomatoes, halved
- 1 large cucumber, halved and sliced
- 1 medium red onion, halved and sliced

Directions

- In a large bowl, combine tomatoes, cucumber, and onion.
- Add vinaigrette and toss to coat.
- Cover properly and Refrigerate.
- Stir in cheese before serving.
- Serve and enjoy.

Greek couscous salad

These veggies are eaten raw as true Mediterranean Sea diet recipe; they are so hearty and delicious.

Ingredients

- ½ cup of olive oil
- ½ cup of crumbled feta cheese
- ¼ cup of lemon juice
- 1 teaspoon of adobo seasoning
- 1-¾ cups of uncooked whole wheat couscous
- 2 cups of grape tomatoes, halved
- 1 can of reduced-sodium chicken broth
- 1 cup of coarsely chopped fresh parsley
- 1-½ teaspoons of grated lemon zest
- ¼ teaspoon of salt
- 1 can of sliced ripe olives, drained
- 1 cucumber, halved lengthwise and sliced
- 4 green onions, chopped

Directions

- In a large saucepan, bring broth to a boil.
- Stir in couscous.

- Remove from heat leave to settle covered to absorb the broth in 5 minutes.
- Transfer to a large bowl let cool totally.
- Whisk all dressing ingredients.
- Add tomatoes, cucumber, olives, parsley, and green onions to couscous
- Stir in the dressing.
- Next, stir in cheese.
- You can either serve immediately or refrigerate.
- Serve cold and enjoy.

Mediterranean shrimp orzo salad

Trust me, this recipe will not fail to stand out on a buffet. It is loaded with abundant shrimp, peppers, olives and artichoke hearts. The components make a real Mediterranean Sea diet with variety of vegetables.

Ingredients

- ¾ cup of Greek vinaigrette
- 1/3 cup of chopped fresh dill
- ¾ pound of peeled and deveined cooked shrimp
- 1 cup of finely chopped green pepper
- 1 package of orzo pasta
- ¾ cup of finely chopped red onion
- ½ cup of pitted Greek olives
- 1 cup of finely chopped sweet red pepper
- ½ cup of minced fresh parsley
- 1 can of water-packed quartered artichoke hearts

Directions

- Cook orzo as directed on the package.

- Drain excess water when ready and rinse with cold water, drain again.
- In a large bowl, combine orzo, vegetables, shrimp, olives, and herbs.
- Add vinaigrette make sure to toss to coat.
- Keep refrigerated when properly covered until serving.
- Enjoy.

Arugula and wild rice salad

This recipe features toasted almond, feta, lemon dressing, dried cherries and of course arugula. It is gluten free and delicious for lunch and dinner.

Ingredients

- ½ cup of sliced almonds
- 5 ounces of arugula
- Freshly ground black pepper,
- 2 teaspoons of Dijon mustard
- ½ cup of coarsely chopped fresh basil
- 1 teaspoon of honey
- ½ cup of crumbled feta
- ½ teaspoon of olive oil
- 2 tablespoons of lemon juice
- 1 cup wild rice, rinsed
- 1 medium clove garlic
- ½ cup of dried tart cherries chopped
- ¼ teaspoon of sea salt

Directions

- Bring a large pot of water to boil.
- Add the rice cook for 20 – 35 minutes.

- Remove, drain the rice and return to pot.
- Cover let simmer for 10 minutes. Then uncover.
- Warm 1 teaspoon of olive oil in a small skillet over medium temperature.
- Add almonds and a pinch of salt let cook until golden and fragrant in 4 – 5 minutes.
- In a small bowl, whisk dressing ingredients until blended.
- Move the cooled rice to a large bowl.
- Add arugula together with chopped basil, sour cherries, almonds, and feta.
- Pour in the dressing, toss and season to taste with pepper.
- Serve and enjoy.

Masala lentil salad with cumin roasted carrots

This recipe is protein rich form the lentils and fresh greens infused with vinaigrette. A typical healthy Mediterranean Sea diet.

Ingredients

- 1 teaspoon garam masala
- 5 tablespoons extra-virgin olive oil
- ½ medium red onion, finely chopped
- 1 tablespoon maple syrup
- 1 ½ teaspoons ground cumin
- Salt and ground black pepper
- Toasted pumpkin seeds
- 2 tablespoons apple cider vinegar
- Ground black pepper
- 1 ½ pounds carrots, peeled and sliced
- 2 cups firmly packed baby arugula
- ⅓ cup chopped fresh mint leaves
- 1 cup dried beluga
- 1 clove garlic, minced
- 1 teaspoon minced ginger

Directions

- Preheat the oven to 400°F.
- Align a baking sheet with parchment paper.
- Place the carrots in a large bowl.
- Drizzle with the oil and maple syrup.
- Sprinkle with cumin, let toss to coat.
- Move to the lined baking sheet make sure to spread in a single layer.
- Season salt and pepper.
- Let bake for 30 – 40 minutes till brown.
- Place the lentils in a pot of water to cover by 4 inches.
- Boil, reduce the heat let simmer for 20 – 30 minutes.
- Drain excess water.
- Place in carrots with lentils in a large bowl let settle for 10 minutes.
- Add arugula, onion, and mint.
- Combine the remaining ingredients in a small bowl whisk to coat.
- Pour the dressing over the salad toss to combined.

- Taste and season accordingly.
- Drizzle with pomegranate molasses.
- Serve and enjoy

Roasted and raw carrot salad with avocado

This recipe reflects the power embedded within herbs. As a result, the carrots are herbed with avocado and mustard dressing. Very delicious for any meal, lunch or dinner.

Ingredients

- Freshly ground black pepper
- 2 tablespoons of extra-virgin olive oil
- Pinch of red pepper flakes
- Salt
- ⅓ cup of torn fresh leafy herbs
- 1 large ripe avocado
- 4 tablespoons of sunshine salad dressing
- ¾ teaspoon of flaky sea salt
- ⅓ cup of chopped green onion
- 2 pounds of carrots

Directions

- Preheat your oven to 425 °F.
- Align a large baking sheet with parchment paper.

- Toss the carrots on the baking sheet with enough olive oil to coat.
- Let bake for 25 – 30 minutes until tender and deeply golden on the edges.
- Place carrot rounds in a bowl filled with water along with a handful of ice cubes. Set aside.
- After roasting carrots, organize them across a platter.
- Drain carrots, sprinkle over the roasted carrots.
- Cut avocado slice half of the avocado, scoop out with a large spoon.
- Arrange over the salad.
- Drizzle the salad dressing lightly across the salad.
- Sprinkle onion and leafy herbs on top.
- Sprinkle with salt, red pepper flakes.
- Serve and enjoy.

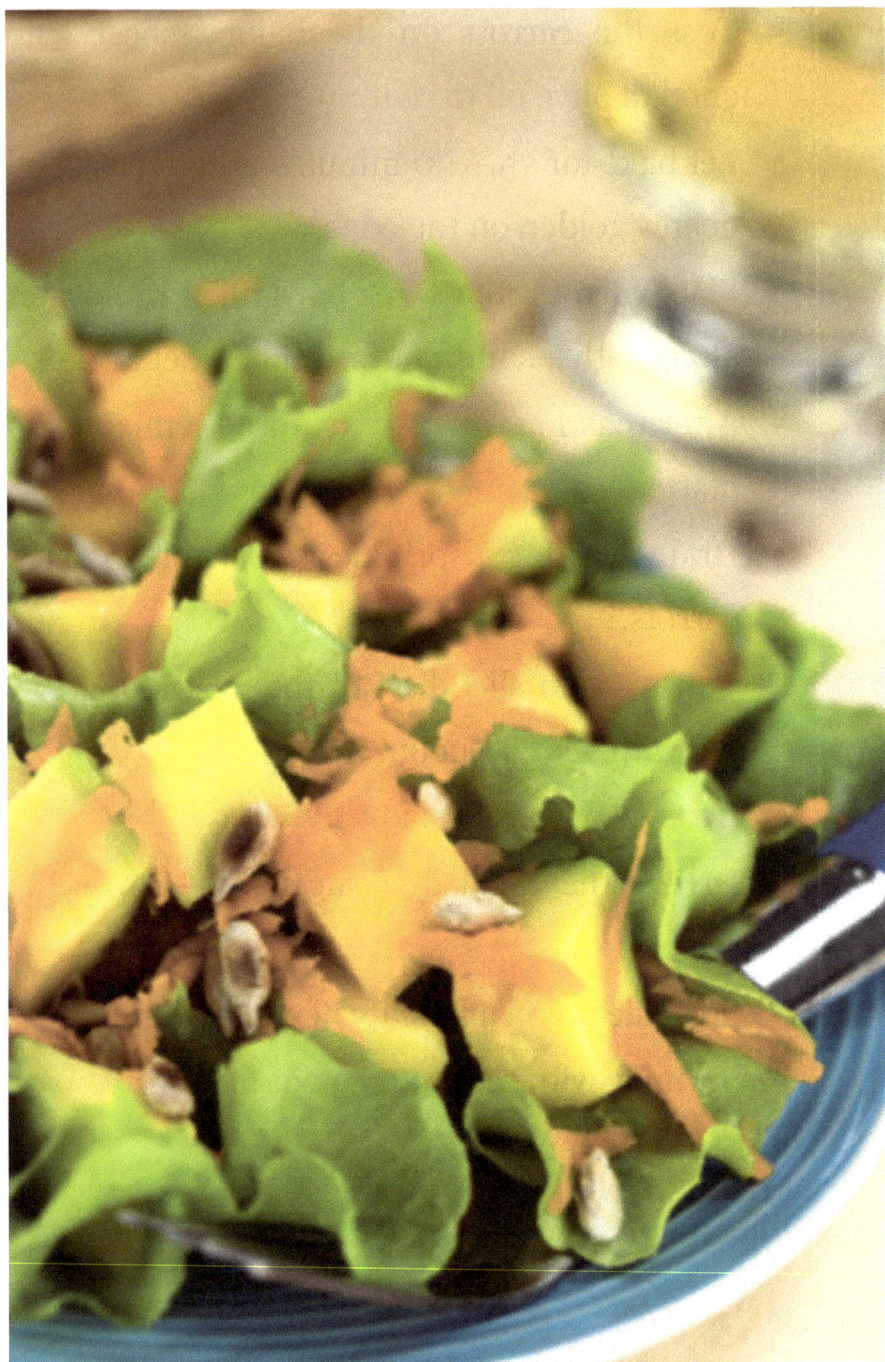

Orange orzo salad with almond, olives, and feta

This particular recipe features wonderfully bright Mediterranean Sea diet flavors. It is prepared with toasted almond, parsley, cucumber and green onions among others listed below.

Ingredients

- ¼ cup of fresh-squeezed orange juice
- ½ cup of raw almonds
- 2 tablespoons of white wine vinegar
- 1 cup of chopped flat-leaf parsley
- ¼ teaspoon of salt
- ¼ cup of extra-virgin olive oil
- 1 medium clove garlic, minced
- ½ cup of pitted Kalamata olives
- ½ cup of chopped green onion
- 8 ounces of whole wheat orzo pasta
- Freshly ground black pepper
- ½ cup of raisins, preferably golden
- ½ cup of crumbled feta cheese

- 1 teaspoon of orange zest

Directions

- Boil salted water in a large pot.
- Add the orzo let cook according to the package Directions.
- Drain and reserve some pasta cooking water.
- Rinse under running water until the orzo cool.
- In a medium skillet over medium heat, toast the almonds keep stirring to attain fragrance and golden color in 5 minutes.
- Move almonds to a cutting board, chop.
- Combine orzo, parsley, chopped almonds, green onion, olives, raisins, and feta in a large bowl.
- Combine orange zest, garlic, olive oil, orange juice, vinegar, and salt in small cup.
- Add ¼ cup of the reserved pasta cooking water, whisk to blended.
- Pour the dressing over the salad, toss to combine.
- Season with pepper accordingly.
- Allow orzo salad rest for 10 minutes or more.

- Again season to taste.
- Serve an enjoy.

Crunchy Thai peanut quinoa salad

Ingredients

- ½ cup chopped cilantro
- ¼ cup thinly sliced green onion
- 1 teaspoon toasted sesame oil
- 1 ½ cups water
- Pinch of red pepper flakes
- ¼ cup roasted and salted peanuts
- 1 teaspoon grated fresh ginger
- ½ lime, juiced
- ¼ cup smooth peanut butter
- ¾ cup uncooked quinoa
- 3 tablespoons tamari
- 1 tablespoon maple syrup
- 1 tablespoon rice vinegar
- 1 cup grated carrot
- 1 cup thinly sliced snow peas
- 2 cups shredded cabbage

Directions

- In a medium-sized pot, combine quinoa and water.

- Boil over medium heat, then reduce lower the heat to simmer all the water is absorbed.
- Take off heat source, cover let sit for 5 minutes. Set aside.
- Whisk the peanut butter and tamari till smooth.
- Add and whisk the remaining ingredients until smooth. Add water if too thick.
- In a large serving bowl, combine the quinoa, carrot, cilantro, shredded cabbage, snow peas, and green onion, toss.
- Introduce peanut sauce, toss again until fully coated.
- Taste and season accordingly.
- Garnish with peanut.
- Serve and enjoy.

Colorful veggie lettuce wraps

This recipe is largely a healthy delicious appetizer or just a light meal. It is vegan with colorful wraps.

Ingredients

- 2 tablespoons of tamari
- 2 heads of butter lettuce
- 3 cups of thinly sliced crisp vegetables
- 2 teaspoons of toasted sesame oil
- ¼ teaspoon of salt
- 4 ½ ounces of soba noodles
- ¾ cup of sliced green onions
- 1 ½ cups of edamame hummus
- ¼ cup of rice vinegar
- 2 tablespoons of sesame seeds

Directions

- Bring a pot of salted water to boil.
- In a medium sized bowl, combine vinegar, vegetables, and salt, toss to combine, then let mixture marinate for 10 minutes.
- Cook the soba noodles as per package instruction.

- Drain, then return them to the pot, place in stir in sesame seeds, onions, tamari, and sesame oil. Set aside.
- Spread hummus over the center of a lettuce leaf.
- Top with bit of soba noodles, pickled veggies.
- Sprinkle lightly with sesame seeds
- Serve and enjoy.

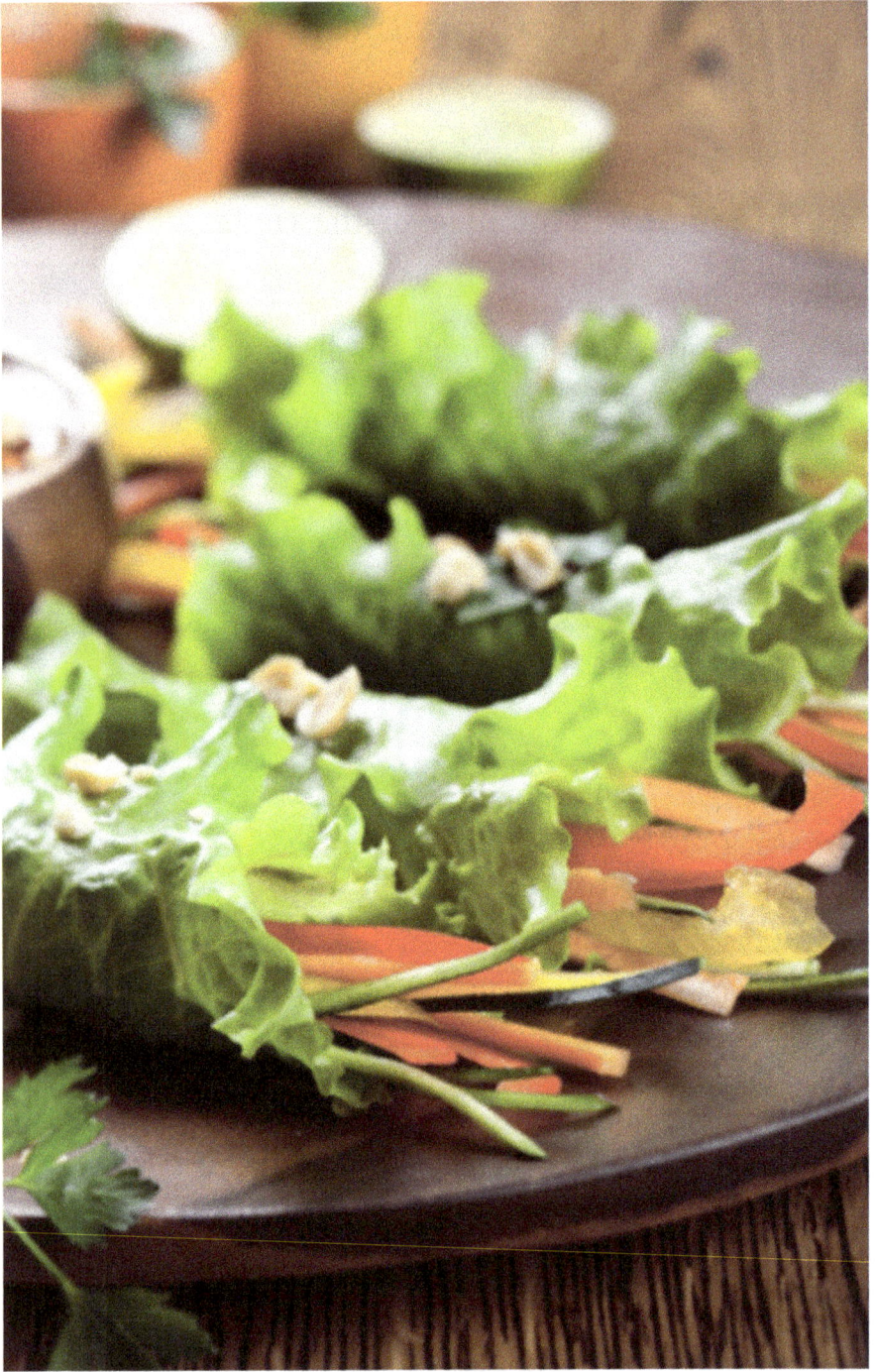

Chicken bacon salad with honey mustard dressing

With a juicy chicken breast, this is a quick easy recipe to make in 20 minutes. The crispy bacon is made together with veggies suitable for vegetarians as the Mediterranean Sea diet agitates. It is a perfect tasty meal for the day, do not miss to try it out with the step by step procedure below.

Ingredients

- Salt & black pepper
- 2 teaspoon of extra virgin olive oil
- ½ small onion, optional
- 4 teaspoon of white wine vinegar
- 1 cup cherry tomatoes
- 8 ounces thin-sliced chicken breasts
- 2 tablespoons of honey
- 2 tablespoons of lemon juice
- ⅓ cup parmesan cheese, grated
- 6 tablespoons of extra virgin olive oil
- 5 ounces of mixed lettuce leaves
- 2 teaspoon of spicy mustard

- [Paprika](#)

Directions

- Fry the bacon in a frying pan.
- Move it onto a plate lined with paper kitchen towel when it is ready fried to get rid of the excess fat.
- Clean the pan of any excess fat then add in the olive oil.
- Season the chicken breasts with salt, pepper and paprika on every side.
- Cook on both sides for 4 minutes or till when ready cooked.
- Cut the cherry tomatoes in halves and slice the onion into rings.
- Divide mixed onion, lettuce leaves, cherry tomatoes in two separate bowls.
- Top with chicken slices, parmesan and bacon.
- Serve and enjoy.

Dad's Greek salad

Salads are a healthy sauce of diet regardless which salad. The dad's Greek salad is distinctive because of the olives, feta, cucumber and tomatoes. The olive oil is used to dress the salad with some vinegar and cheese as indicated below.

Ingredients

- 3 tablespoons of red wine vinegar
- ¼ cup of olive oil
- 4 large tomatoes coarsely cup and seeds removed
- 2 cups of thinly sliced cucumbers
- A small red onion cut into two and thinly sliced
- ¼ teaspoon of salt
- 1/8 teaspoon of pepper
- ¼ teaspoon of dried oregano (this is option)
- ¾ cup of pitted Greek olives
- ¾ cup of crumbled feta cheese

Directions

- Place all the cucumbers, onion, tomatoes in one large bowl at once.

- Get a small bowl to whisk oil, vinegar, pepper, oregano, and salt
- Blend until it is finely blended.
- Drizzle over salad and toast it to coat.
- Then fill the top with olives and cheese
- Serve and enjoy

Tzatziki potato salad

Ingredients

- 2 tablespoons snipped fresh dill
- 1 carton (12 ounces) refrigerated tzatziki sauce
- 2 celery ribs, thinly sliced
- 2 tablespoons minced fresh parsley
- ¼ teaspoon celery salt
- 3 pounds small red potatoes, halved
- 2 green onions, chopped
- ½ cup plain Greek yogurt
- ¼ teaspoon pepper
- ½ teaspoon salt
- 1 tablespoon minced fresh mint, optional

Directions

- Place the potatoes in an oven; preferably a Dutch oven.
- Cover the potatoes with water then bring to boil.
- Continue to cook over reduced heat for about 10 – 15 minutes until tender.
- Drain the excess water and cool completely.

- Mix the tzatziki sauce, yogurt, celery, dill, parsley, salt, green onions, pepper, and celery salt in a smaller bowl.
- Spoon over the cooked potatoes then toss to coat.
- Refrigerate while covered until cold.
- Serve and enjoy

Mediterranean cobb salad

The Mediterranean cobb salad are classic diet, mainly when there is a flair added to it. The ingredients and instruction are listed below.

Ingredients

- ½ cup of sour cream or plain yogurt
- ¼ cup of milk
- 1 package of falafel mix (6 ounces)
- ¼ cup of chopped seeded peeled cucumber
- ½ cup of pitted finely chopped Greek olives
- 8 cups of bacon strips, cooked and crumbled
- 2 medium sized finely seeded and chopped tomatoes
- 1 medium ripe peeled and chopped avocado
- 3 hard boiled large chopped eggs
- 4 cups of baby spinach
- 4 cups of torn romaine
- ¼ teaspoon of salt
- 1 teaspoon of minced parsley

Directions

- Cook the falafel depending on the manufacturer's Directions.
- Let it cool off
- Crumble and or coarsely chop falafel
- Combine the sour cream, cucumber, parsley, salt and milk in a small bowl
- In a separate larger bowl, combine spinach and romaine.
- Transfer to a platter
- Organize the crumbled falafel and the remaining ingredients over greens
- Drizzle with dressing ready for serving

Nectarine and beet salad

This recipe makes a scrumptious inclusion to variety of mixed greens mainly with the beets, nectarines and feta cheese. The choice of ingredients may not reflect your favorite salad but that is a lie of one's eyes. This salad can become your favorite choice for a home salad.

Ingredients

- ½ cup of crumbled feta cheese
- ½ of medium sized sliced nectarines
- 1 can of sliced drained beets (14 – ½ ounces)
- 2 packages of spring greens mixed salad (5 ounces each)
- ½ cup of balsamic vinaigrette

Directions

- Toss all greens in a serving dish with nectarine and vinaigrette
- Top with cheese and the beets
- Serve immediately for a better taste

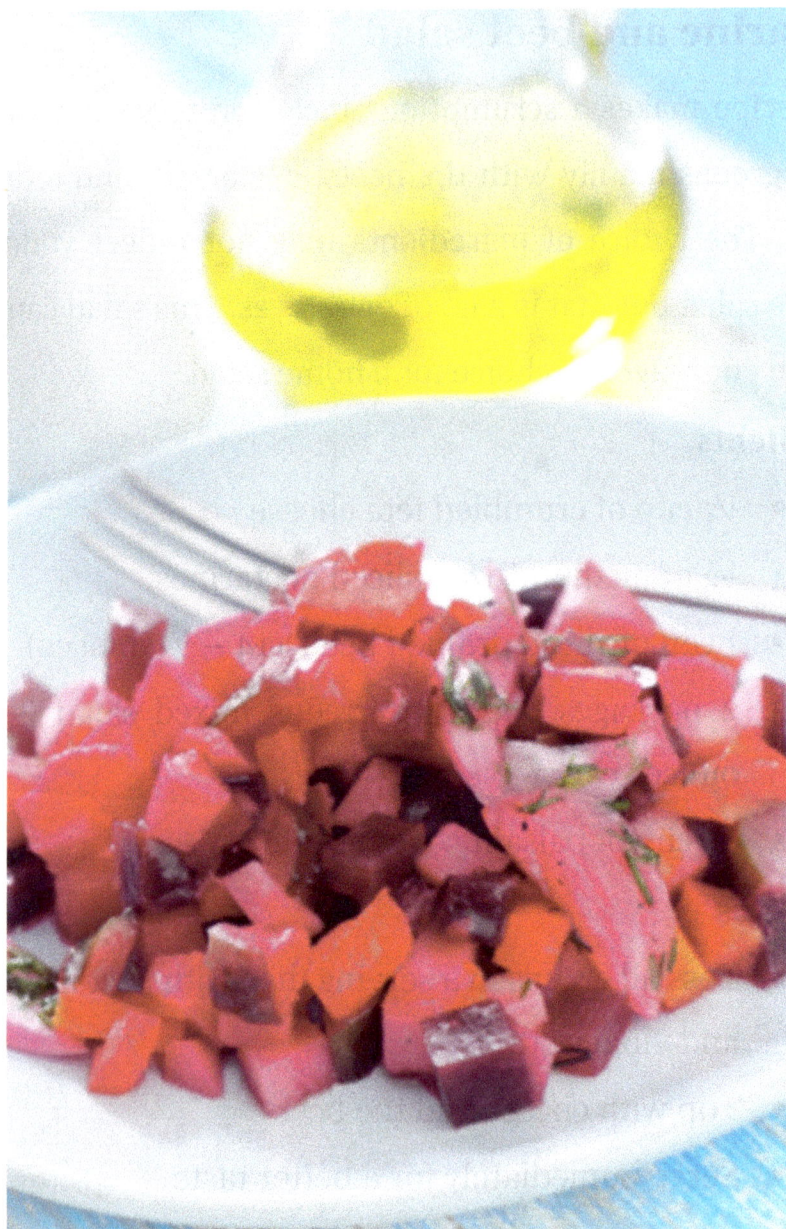

Balsamic cucumber salad

Cucumber is a perfect healthy salad for variety of dishes especially for kabobs, chicken and or anything hot off the grill. The Directions and directions are shown below.

Ingredients

- ½ cup of balsamic vinaigrette
- 1 medium halved and thinly sliced red onions
- 1 large halved and sliced cucumber
- 2 cups of grape tomatoes cut into half

Directions

- Combine the tomatoes, onions, cucumber in a large bowl
- Introduce vinaigrette then toss to coat.
- Refrigerate when it is cover until serving
- Stir in the cheese and then serve with a slotted spoon
- Enjoy

Tzatziki shrimp cucumber rounds

Ingredients

- 2 tablespoons of finely chopped peeled cucumber
- 2 medium size cucumbers slices cut into ¼ -in
- 1.4 cup of reduced fat plain yogurt
- 1/8 teaspoon of garlic salt
- 6 bacon strips
- 1/8 teaspoon of dill weed
- 1 or 2 tablespoons of canola oil
- 24 shrimp peeled and deveined (32 – 40 pound)

Instruction

- Combine the yogurt, garlic salt, dill and chopped cucumber to set aside in a small bowl.
- Lengthwise and widthwise, evenly cut each bacon in halves.
- Using the bacon, wrap each piece of shrimp and lock them with a toothpick.
- In a larger nonstick skillet, heat the oil with medium temperature.

- Cook the shrimp in manageable batches for 3 – 4 minutes on every side until crispy
- Spoon the yogurt sauce on each cucumber slice.
- Top with the shrimp
- Serve and enjoy

Tomato feta salad

This recipe is perfect for balsamic dressing. It can be topped and served with a variety of dishes or even combined with other veggies to quench the appetite for fresh healthy vegetables. Below are the ingredients and Directions.

Ingredients

- 2 tablespoons of balsamic vinegar
- ¼ cup of crumbles feta cheese
- 1 – ¼ teaspoon of minced basil (fresh or dried)
- ½ teaspoon of salt
- ½ cup of coarsely chopped sweet onions
- 1 pound of grape or cherry tomatoes
- 2 tablespoon of olive oil

Directions

- Using a larger bowl, combine the basil, salt, and vinegar.
- Introduce the onion then toss to coat.
- Let it settle for 5 minutes.
- Introduce the tomatoes, feta cheese, and oil and toss to coat.

- Serve and enjoy

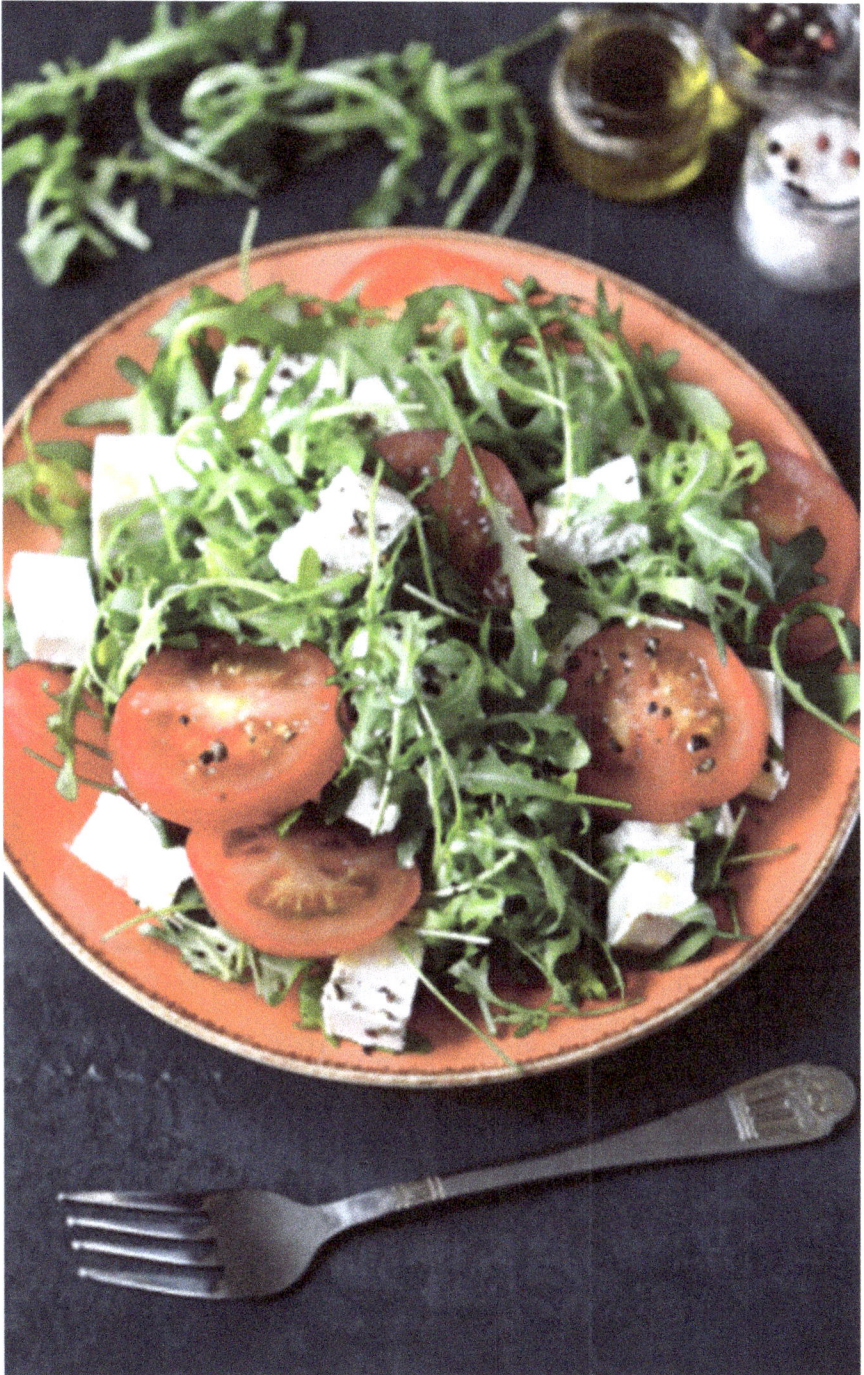

Cherry tomato salad

This very recipe emerged from the need and urgency to use bumper crops of delicious cherry tomatoes commonly grown. Since then, the ingredients and directions below have been used to utilize cherry tomatoes.

Ingredients

- 1 or 2 teaspoons of minced oregano
- ¼ cup of canola oil
- ¼ cup of minced parsley
- ½ teaspoon of salt
- ½ teaspoon of sugar
- 1 quart of cherry tomatoes
- 3 tablespoons of white vinegar
- 1 teaspoon of minced basil

Directions

- In a shallow bowl, place all the tomatoes.
- In another small bowl, mix whisk oil, salt, sugar, and vinegar until evenly blended.
- Stir in the herbs.
- Pour the over tomatoes gently to toss and coat.
- Cover and refrigerate overnight.

- Serve and enjoy

Greek salad dressing

Ingredients

- ½ teaspoon of dried oregano
- ¼ teaspoon of pepper
- ½ cup of olive oil
- ½ teaspoon of salt
- ¼ cup of red wine vinegar
- 2 minced garlic cloves
- 1 teaspoon of Dijon mustard
- 2 teaspoons of lemon juice

Directions

- In a tight fitting lid jar, combine all the ingredients at once.
- Shake well until fully blended.
- Serve and enjoy.

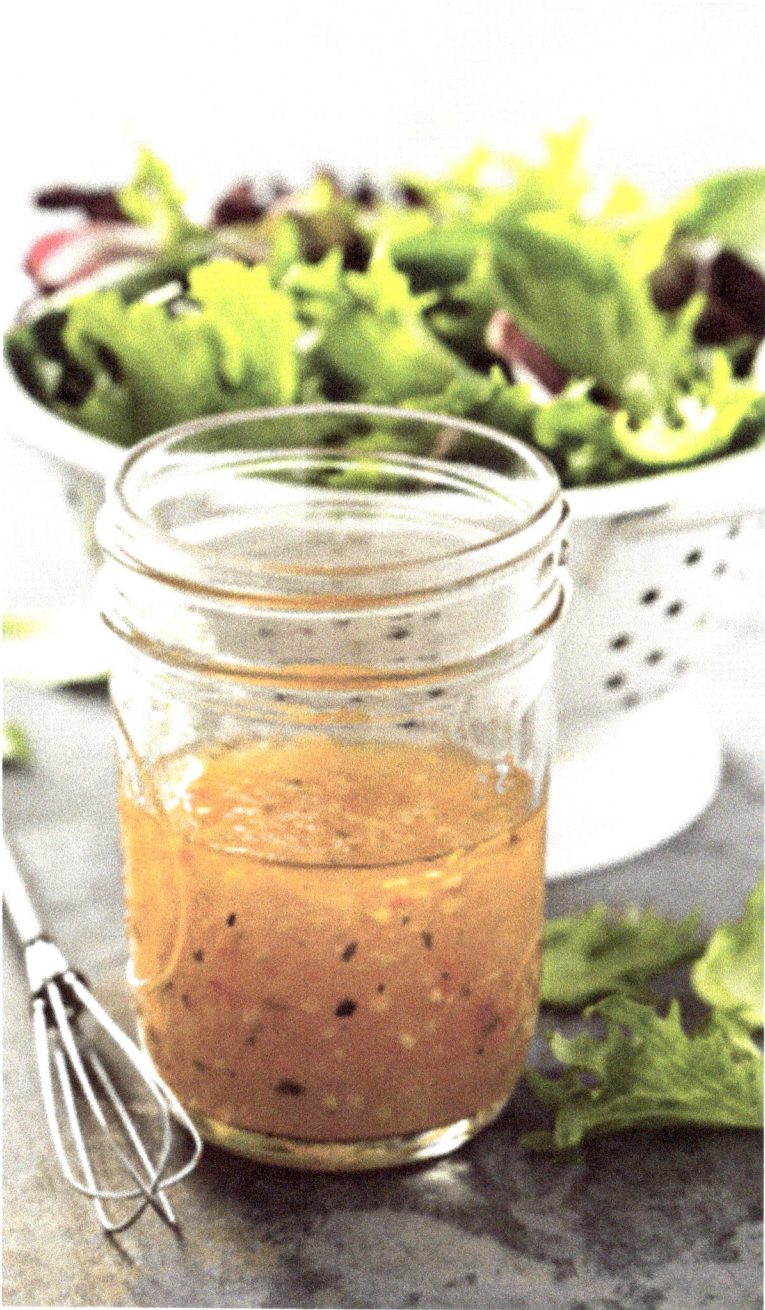

Garden tomato salad

One can make this garden tomato recipe conveniently at any time as long as they have a garden of fresh tomatoes. The nourishing looks of a fresh tomato makes this a perfect salad for a Mediterranean Sea diet.

Ingredients

- ¼ cup of olive oil
- ½ teaspoon of salt
- 2 tablespoons of cider vinegar
- 1 minced garlic clove
- 1 teaspoon of minced chives
- 1 teaspoon of minced basil
- 1 large sweet onions cut into wedges
- 3 large tomatoes cut into wedges
- 1 large sliced cucumber

Directions

- Combine cucumber, tomatoes, and onions in a large bowl.
- In another small bowl, whisk the dressing ingredients until uniformly blended (the

remaining ingredients apart from tomatoes, cucumber, and onions)

- Drizzle over the salad then slowly toss to coat.
- Serve immediately or store under refrigeration if need be.

White bean salad

This recipe includes the preparation of white beans loaded with Mediterranean Sea diet flavors. Unlike other recipes, this one does not involve fancy dressing; as such, it is only lemon juice and extra virgin oil that is important.

Ingredients

- 1 cup chopped fresh parsley
- 4 green onions, chopped
- 1 English cucumber, diced
- 10 orzo grape or cherry tomatoes, halved
- Feta cheese, optional
- Salt and pepper
- 2 cans of rinsed and drained white beans
- 15 to 20 mint leaves, chopped
- 1 lemon, zested and juiced
- Extra virgin olive oil
- 1 teaspoon of Za'atar
- ½ teaspoon of Sumac and Aleppo .

Directions

- In a large bowl, combine the tomatoes, green onions, mint, cucumber, beans, and parsley.

- Proceed to add lemon zest.
- Season with pepper and salt.
- Add the za'atar, Aleppo pepper, and sumac.
- Finish up the recipe with lemon juice which can be drizzled with 2 or 3 tablespoon of extra virgin olive oil.
- Do a thorough toss to let combine.
- Adjust the season according to the taste.
- Introduce the feta cheese, if desired.
- Allow the salad to settle in the dressing for 30 – 31 minutes just before serving
- Serve.

3-ingredient Mediterranean salad

Ingredients

- 1 teaspoon of ground Sumac
- salt
- 2 teaspoons of freshly squeezed lemon juice
- 1 Large diced cucumber
- ½ to ¾ packed cup/ 15 to 20 g chopped fresh parsley leaves
- ½ teaspoon of black pepper
- 2 teaspoon of Early Harvest extra virgin olive oil
- 6 diced Roma tomatoes

Directions

- Put the diced tomatoes, parsley in a larger salad bowl.
- Add salt and set aside for approximately 4 minutes
- Add all remaining ingredients and toss the salad gently.
- Give the flavors some minutes to melt before serving.
- Enjoy

Traditional Greek salad

Ingredients

- 1 English cucumber partially peeled making a striped pattern
- ½ teaspoon of dried oregano
- Blocks of Greek feta cheese do not crumble the feta, leave it in large pieces
- Greek pitted Kalamata olives a handful to your liking
- 4 teaspoon of quality extra virgin olive oil
- 1 medium red onion
- kosher salt a pinch
- 4 Medium juicy tomatoes
- 1-2 teaspoon of red wine vinegar
- 1 green bell pepper cored

Instruction

- Begin by cutting the red onions into halves, then slice into crescent moon shape.
- Cut the tomatoes into wedges or even you can slice others in rounds.
- Cut the cucumber into half and slice into halves.

- The bell pepper should be sliced into rings.
- Combine all the ingredients in the above steps in a large salad dish.
- Add some pitted Kalamata olives.
- Using kosher salt, season lightly with some dried oregano.
- Pour wine vinegar and olive oil all over the salad.
- Toss gently to combine and blend. Be sure not to over mix.
- Introduce the feta block right on top and sprinkle with more of the dried oregano.
- Serve with crusty bread and enjoy.

Mediterranean watermelon salad

Watermelon a special healthy gift to the kidney can be used to make a perfect salad using only three main ingredients typically watermelon, feta cheese, cucumber. Adding fresh mint, honey vinaigrette, and basil propels this recipe to a whole new horizon.

Ingredients

- ½ peeled watermelon cut in cubes
- ½ cup of crumble feta cheese
- 15 fresh chopped mint leaves
- 15 chopped fresh basil leaves
- 1 cucumber
- 2 teaspoon of extra virgin olive oil
- 2 tablespoons of honey
- 2 teaspoons of lime juice
- Pinch of salt

Directions

- Whisk the honey together with olive oil, pinch of salt, and lime juice.
- Keep the mixture aside for a while.
- In a large bowl, serve the platter with sides.

- Combine the cucumber, fresh herbs, and watermelon together.
- Top the salad with honey vinaigrette and toss to allow massive combination.
- Top with feta cheese
- Sever and enjoy.

Mediterranean chickpea salad

Ingredients

- 1 large thinly sliced eggplant
- Salt
- oil for frying
- 1 cup cooked or canned chickpeas
- 3 tablespoons of Za'atar spice , divided
- 3 Roma tomatoes, diced
- ½ diced English cucumber, diced
- 1 small red onion, sliced in ½ moons
- 1 cup chopped parsley
- 1 cup chopped dill
- 1-2 garlic cloves, minced
- 1 large lime, juice of
- ⅓ cup Early Harvest extra virgin olive oil
- Salt and Pepper

Directions

- Place the eggplants on a tray large enough to accommodate them, then sprinkle with salt.
- Allow it to settle for 30 minutes.

- Introduce another large tray or baking sheet with paper bags topped with paper towel.
- Place it near the stove.
- Heat about 4 tablespoons of extra virgin oil after patting the eggplants dry over a medium temperature to a point of simmering.
- Fry the eggplants in batches in the oil. Ensure not to crowd the skillet.
- After the eggplants have turned golden brown on every side, remove and arrange them on a paper towel-lined tray to allowing draining and cooling.
- Assemble the eggplants on a serving dish and sprinkle with 1 tablespoon of za'atar.
- In a medium sized mixing bowl, combine the cucumbers, chickpeas, parsley, red onions, tomatoes, and the dill.
- Add the remaining za'atar and stir gently
- In a separate small bowl, whisk the dressing together.
- Drizzle 2 tablespoons of the salad dressing over the already fried eggplants.

- The remaining dressing should be poured over the chickpeas salad mix.
- Add the chickpea salad to the eggplant in a serving dish.
- Enjoy.

Chicken sharwarma salad bowls

Ingredients

- ¾ tablespoon of garlic powder
- Salt
- ¾ tablespoon of paprika
- ¾ tablespoon of ground coriander
- 8 boneless, skinless chicken thighs
- ¾ tablespoon of ground cumin
- ½ teaspoon of ground cloves
- ½ teaspoon of cayenne pepper
- ¾ tablespoon of turmeric powder
- ⅓ cup extra virgin olive oil
- 1 large onion, thinly sliced
- 1 large lemon, juice of
- 1 garlic clove minced
- 8 oz. baby arugula
- 2 to 3 Roma tomatoes, diced
- Sumac approximately ½ teaspoon
- Juice of 1 lemon
- Extra Virgin Olive Oil
- ¼ red onion, thinly sliced

- 1 English cucumber, diced
- Salt and pepper

Directions

- In a small bowl, mix majority of the ingredients typically the coriander, turmeric, cumin, garlic power, paprika, and cloves.
- Keep the sharwarma spice for later
- Pat the chicken thighs dry and season with salt on both sides.
- Then thinly slice into small bite-sized pieces.
- Put the chicken in a large bowl, then add the shawarma spices, then toss to coat.
- Introduce the onions, olive oil, and lemon juice.
- Toss everything together to combine, then set aside as you prepare the salad
- Cover totally for refrigeration for up to 3 hours. If there is time for you to wait, refrigerate overnight.
- Prepare the salad in a mixing bowl by combining the tomatoes, cucumbers, arugula, and onions over a medium temperature.

- In a separate small bowl combine the olive oil, garlic, pepper, salt, sumac, and lemon juice to make the dressing, blend thoroughly well.
- Pour the dressing over the salad and toss to let combine.
- Heat another extra virgin olive oil in a large skillet over medium temperature until when it simmers without smoke.
- Add the chicken and let cook for 5 – 6 minutes.
- Toss and continue to cook for another 5 – 6 minute until when the chicken is ready.
- Divide the salad into serving dishes, then add the ready cooked chicken sharwarma.
- Serve and enjoy with pit wedges if desired.

Mediterranean couscous salad

This salad recipe is yet loaded with flavorful and highly nutritious from sources such as fresh herbs, chickpeas, zippy lemon dill vinaigrette. Other than that, the dish is famous for its versatility for lunch, supper and or breakfast. Interestingly, it can be made ahead of time before hunger hunts you down.

Ingredients

- 15-20 fresh basil leaves, roughly chopped or torn
- Water
- 1 tsp dill weed
- 15 ounces can chickpeas
- 2 cups Pearl Couscous
- salt and pepper
- Private Reserve extra virgin olive oil
- 1 large lemon, juice of
- 14 ounces can artichoke hearts
- ⅓ cup extra virgin olive oil
- ½ English cucumber, chopped
- 2 cups grape tomatoes, halved

- ½ cup pitted Kalamata olive
- ⅓ cup finely chopped red onions
- 1 to 2 garlic cloves, minced
- 3 ounces of fresh baby mozzarella optional

Directions

- Place all the vinaigrette ingredients in a bowl to make the lemon-dill vinaigrette.
- Whisk together to combine keep aside for a short while.
- In a medium-sized pot, heat two tablespoons of [olive oil](#) .
- Briefly, Sauté the couscous in the olive oil to turn golden brown.
- Add boiling water about 3 cups or as instructed to cook the couscous.
- Drain excess water in a colander when ready and also keep aside in a bowl allow to cool.
- Combine all the remaining ingredients except the basil and mozzarella in a large mixing bowl.
- Add the couscous and the basil and mix together gently

- It is time to give the lemon-dill vinaigrette a quick whisk, also add to the couscous salad.
- Mix again to combine.
- Test and adjust the salt accordingly.
- Lastly, mix in the mozzarella cheese and garnish with more fresh basil.
- Serve and enjoy.

Mediterranean cauliflower salad

Ingredients

- [Extra virgin olive oil](#)
- 1 whole bunch of parsley, stems partially removed
- Kosher salt and pepper
- 1 English cucumber chopped
- ½ red onion, chopped
- 1 head raw cauliflower, cut into florets
- 1 to 2 garlic cloves, minced
- 3 – 4 Roma tomatoes, chopped
- Juice of 2 lemons

Directions

- In a bowl of a food processor fitted with a blade, put the cauliflower florets.
- Pulse briefly until the cauliflower turns rice-like in texture.
- Move chopped cauliflower into a larger bowl.
- Add the parsley, cucumbers, tomatoes, and onions let toss to combine.
- Add minced garlic and season with salt and pepper.

- Add fresh lemon juice and drizzle with extra virgin olive oil.
- Toss once again to combine.
- Keep the cauliflower salad aside for some minutes let soften and absorb dressing.
- Serve and enjoy.

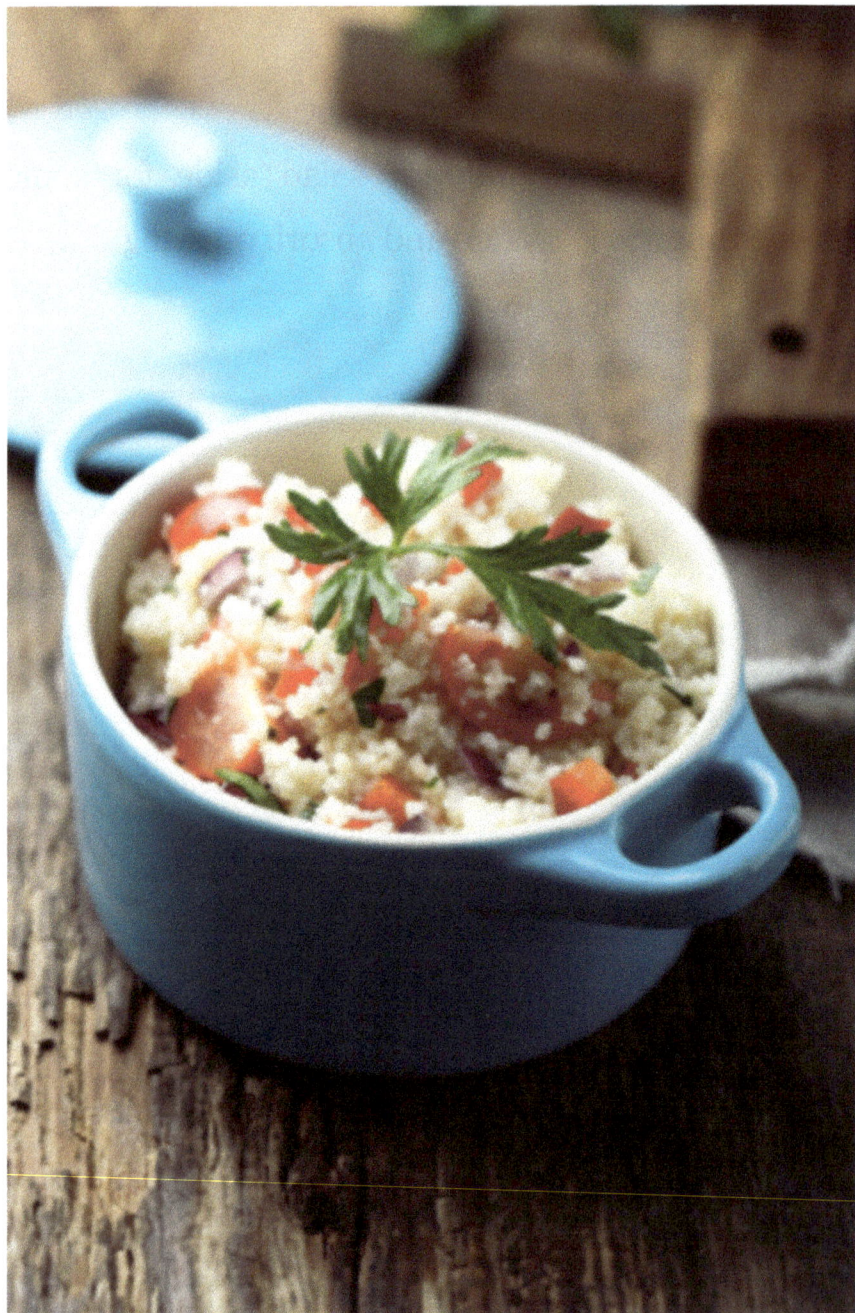

Watermelon cups

This recipe is largely and appetizer pretty and sweet to enjoy. In addition, watermelon is a gift to the kidney which boosts its functionality. The watermelon cut into cubes hold with a refreshing topping that shows red onions, fresh herbs and cucumber brings out a person's appetite to eat them.

Ingredients

- 15 – 17 watermelon cubes without seeds
- 5 teaspoons of red onions finely chopped
- 2 teaspoons of mint freshly minced
- 1/3 cups of chopped cucumber
- 2 teaspoons of fresh cilantro minced
- ½ teaspoon of lime juice

Directions

- In a watermelon baller, measure spoon, scoop the watermelon blossoms form the center of the cubes.
- Do not totally remove the center of the watermelon, leave about 1/4 in

- Mix all the remaining ingredients in a separate small bowl
- Spoon it into watermelon cubes
- Serve and enjoy your watermelon cups for a healthy kidney

Simple green juice

15 minutes is all it takes to make this handful 6 ingredients healthy juice with its refreshing tast

Ingredients

- 5 celery stalks, ends trimmed
- Handful fresh parsley, 1 ounce
- 1 Inch piece of fresh peeled ginger
- 1 bunch kale, 5 ounces
- ½ large English cucumber
- 1 Granny smith apple

Directions

- Prep all the vegetables after washing.
- Add all the ingredients into a juicer and blend at once.
- Pour the green juice to glasses and serve immediately.
- Enjoy.

Mixed beery smoothie

If you do not like chopping of ingredient, then this is a perfect Mediterranean smoothie you can go for. It gets ready in only 5 minutes. All you need is to blend all the ingredients at once.

Ingredients

- ⅛ cup honey
- ⅓ cup [Greek yogurt](Greek%20yogurt)
- 2 ripe bananas
- 2 cups frozen mixed berry
- 1 cup milk

Directions

- In a blender, combine bananas together with the, frozen berry mix, milk, Greek yogurt, and honey.
- Blend until finely smooth.
- Serve and enjoy.

Apple pear ginger smoothie

This is a dairy free recipe with variety of fruits and ginger as a flavor. It is rich with antioxidants and vitamins from the 5 ingredients.

Ingredients

- 1½ cup of apple juice
- ½ cup rolled oats
- 1 thumb-size ginger, finely grated
- 3 pears cored and diced
- 3 apples preferably red, peeled and diced

Directions

- Process the oats until they are powdery in a food processor.
- Add the remaining ingredients, process until smooth
- Serve and enjoy immediately.

Detox green juice

Among the Mediterranean Sea diet recipes, detox green juice is a perfect immunity booster and a body cleanser. It takes 10 minutes to prepare.

Ingredients

- ½ small lemon, juice only
- 7 ounces of fresh kale
- ½ English of cucumber
- 3 large green apples
- 1 cup fresh spinach

Directions

- Cut the apples into quarters, kale, and cucumber pieces
- Using a juicer, juice everything else apart from the lemon.
- Taste and adjust accordingly with lemon.
- Serve and enjoy.

699. Mango kale smoothie

A combination of mango and kale (herb) makes a wonderful healthy smoothie packed with vitamins and antioxidants.

Ingredients

- 2 tablespoons of honey
- 1 medium banana, cut into chunks
- ½ cup of Greek yogurt
- 1 cup of frozen mango pieces
- 2 cups of chopped kale leaves
- 1 cup of milk

Directions

- Combine every ingredient into a blender.
- Blend until it becomes smooth.
- Transfer into a glass.
- Serve and enjoy.

Matcha iced tea

Matcha iced tea is a perfect Mediterranean Sea diet for a refreshing drink with mint and a ton of flavors.

Ingredients

- 1 lime
- 1 cup of crushed ice
- 2 teaspoon of matcha powder
- 2 cups of cold water
- 5 tablespoon of maple syrup
- 1/4 cup of hot water
- 3 sprigs of fresh mint

Directions

- Combine and mix matcha powder in water in a small dish, mix.
- Place in crushed ice, cold water together with fresh mint in a blender.
- Add in the matcha tea blend briefly for 1 minute.
- Drain.
- Add juice and maple syrup after half of the time has run up.

- Garnish with mint leaves and lime.
- Serve and enjoy.

Mediterranean green salad

This recipe is a perfect outdoor or entertainment recipe or grill parties. It only takes 10 minutes.

Ingredients

- 1 butter lettuce
- 2 tablespoons of honey
- A few fresh mint leaves
- 1 tablespoon of lemon juice
- 2 spring onions
- 2 cups of fresh sweet peas
- 2 green peppers
- 1½ cup cherry tomatoes
- 5 tablespoons of extra virgin olive oil
- 1 cup of mange tout

Directions

- Cut lettuce into thin strips
- Shell the peas.
- Slice the spring onions.
- Cut green peppers into thin strips.
- Half the tomatoes.

- Combine all the ingredients i.e. olive oil, chopped mint leaves. lemon juice, and honey.
- Pour over the salad.
- Serve and enjoy.

Strawberry salad with poppy seeds dressing

This recipe is a typical side dish for a BBQ combined with strawberries, spring onions and lettuce. It gets ready in only 10 minutes.

Ingredients

- 1 tablespoon of balsamic reduction
- 4 tablespoons of [extra virgin olive oil](#)
- 2 cups of fresh strawberries
- 2 tablespoons of poppy seeds
- 1 head of butter lettuce
- 2 spring onions

Directions

- Clean and chop the ingredients and place them in a serving dish.
- Mix them together with hands.
- Combine extra virgin olive oil, poppy seeds, and balsamic reduction. Mix well in a jar.
- Pour the mixture over the salad.
- Serve and enjoy immediately.

.

www.ingramcontent.com/pod-product-compliance
Lightning Source LLC
Chambersburg PA
CBHW062117040426
42336CB00041B/1786